Future Focused Parents-To-Be:
Planning Beyond the Birth

By Kira Dorrian, CHt, HBCE

Copyright © 2018 Kira Dorrian
All rights reserved

DEDICATION

For Guido.

"i carry your heart with me (i carry it in my heart)"
— E.E. Cummings

CONTENTS

Acknowledgements	i
Introduction	1
Avoiding the "Winging It" Approach	4
How to Use This Book	7
Section One: Family Values	9
Section Two: The First Few Months	40
Section Three: All the Months Thereafter	72
Conclusion	93

ACKNOWLEDGEMENTS

I am forever grateful to Mel and Randy DePaoli, and Emma and Jake Berendes, who were my guinea pigs before this book was even a book. A special thanks to all of the couples who then trialed this workbook and gave feedback. And thanks goes to Jennifer Christison the brainstorming and breadsticks that sparked this idea in the first place.

So much gratitude to Noah Bell-Cruz (www.bellboycreative.com) for all of his incredible design work on every project I bring his way, especially this one. An enormous thank you to my copyeditor, Yassmeen Angarola, who spent her last months of pregnancy working on this book. And a huge shout-out to Tracy Barrett Adams for helping with the publishing of this book, and, more importantly, for being such an important part of my creative journey since TBATST were born.

Thanks to Deana Thayer for never running scared when I say "I have an idea" and for inspiring me, always, to be the best Mom I can be. The utmost love and gratitude goes to my beautiful TBATST who rocked my world and then became my muse. And finally, a huge thanks to my husband, David, for saying "that sounds like a great idea" when I said I wanted to write a book.

INTRODUCTION

I had some choice words for my OB when I found out I was expecting twins. To say that I was surprised would be the understatement of the century. To say I was terrified is a close second. You see, I am a planner and let me tell you that two babies at the same time was not in my plan. So, I made lists. A million lists. I had a list for the nursery, a list of books to read, a list of classes to take—you get the idea.

The problem is I didn't make the right lists. I didn't list my priorities, either for myself or for my marriage. I didn't list my family values or the attributes I wished to foster in my two babies. I didn't make those lists because I didn't know I needed them.

And so, my own transition was incredibly challenging. I can only describe it as feeling sucker punched. I was so prepared for my birth, and not at all prepared for what came afterward. I wished that someone had sat me down and helped me set up a plan for success, including helping me set realistic expectations for myself, for my partner, and for my new life as a mother.

This book was written so that YOU won't feel sucker punched. After I finally settled into motherhood it became my life's mission to help parents feel as prepared as possible for their transition into parenthood.

These days many couples go into parenthood with eyes wide open. They've seen their friends struggle. They know it's going to be hard. They know what they don't want to do. But what do they *want* to do? What will they need? And, more importantly, how do they meet their goals and fulfill their needs?

This book will ask you the big questions and help you make the right lists so that when things get hard, you have a foundation and a framework to reference and remind you of what you do want to achieve for yourselves as individuals, as a couple, and as parents.

This book will also help you discover the parenting style that is right for you, list your top five to ten family values, and discuss what steps you need to take together as parents to achieve these goals. It will also help you talk about your needs—both as individuals and as a couple—that might be compromised by having a baby. You have probably already seen your friends struggle with this (heck, that's why you are reading this book!). Some of them fight all the time, or one sleeps all night while the other is up with the baby. Or you may have a friend who never showers anymore and you silently pray when you hang out with her that you won't be *that* mom.

You don't have to be. This book will help you make a plan for when you shower. It sounds silly, I know, but trust me, you need a plan for showering. You will plan for couple time, for how to stay connected, and for ways to avoid becoming only task oriented. You will plan for sick days, for boundary setting, and for a host of other things that will allow you to be the best team possible and to minimize feeling resentful, frustrated, and overwhelmed.

And best of all, you will learn how to be flexible with this plan, so that you aren't locked into anything and can tweak and perfect things along the way.

The best book I read when I was pregnant was so short I finished it in an afternoon. It had all the information I needed without too much fluff, allowing me to get back to the important stuff, like decorating the nursery. The goal of this workbook is to offer something just as quick and easy as my favorite parenting book, so that you can prepare as a couple for the life changes a little one will bring, and then get back to the fun stuff like decorating the nursery or going out for dinner (because you should do as much of that as you can right now).

Parenting is not one-size-fits-all. There isn't a right or wrong way to do it, only what is right or wrong for your family. Figuring out what your core values are and discussing how to meet your core needs together and individually will set you up for success as parents and as a family.

AVOIDING THE "WINGING IT APPROACH"

Here is what I already know about you, simply because you are reading this book:

1. You care about your relationship.
2. You care about your baby and doing right by them.
3. You are likely thinking beyond your birthing day hoping to set yourself up, as best you can, for a successful transition into parenthood.

Well, congratulations! By simply choosing to do a little planning and being intentional as you move into parenthood you are already leagues ahead of the couples who are "planning" to "wing it".

As my partner at Future Focused Parenting, Deana Thayer, says, "Parenting should be the thing you do most on purpose in your life." Unfortunately, too often parents choose the "wing it" approach and get very lost along the way.

Please don't get me wrong, the best laid plans won't always come to fruition, and flexibility is an absolute *necessity* in parenthood, but the bottom line is that having some kind of plan and framework can only set you up for more success, because you have a sense of what you want to achieve.

Think of it this way: if you want to paint a picture you don't just slap paint on a canvas and hope that it ultimately looks like a flower. Instead you set an *intention* to paint a flower and then what that journey looks like can be as creative and unique as you are.

Ok, so some of you are probably thinking "but what about those painters who *do* just slap paint on a canvas as their art follows their emotions?" To that I say, "Yup, that's true!" But please don't forget that they've spent years painting, studying painting, doing all different types of painting and now they are expressing themselves in this way *by choice, with intention,* based on their past experiences as painters. The bottom line is that it is still intentional.

So, with that in mind, would you sit down to paint your very first picture and slap the paint on the canvas hoping that it looks like *something* by the time you were done? Or would you instead choose to paint something and work toward that goal, with as much flexibility and fluidity as needed along the way?

And what if I upped the game? What if I said this painting was also going to be the most important thing you would ever create in your life? This painting has the power to shape the world. It is your *legacy*. How does "winging it" sound now?

The problem with the "winging it" approach to parenthood is that parenthood is, well, *hard.* You've never done it before and you are learning on the job. And parenting requires the kind of quick, on-your-feet thinking of an international spy, so the idea that you can "wing" something that high stakes seems kind of silly.

The other issue that arises with the "winging it" approach is that you and your partner are going to come across situations where you disagree. If there is no cornerstone for your family value system, no plan for how you want to raise this little person, those disagreements have no framework within which to be resolved.

So, let's all agree that parenting should happen with some kind of intentional framework. And truthfully, that can be whatever you want it to be. There isn't a right or a wrong way, but *please* pick *a* way.

It is my intention that this book will help you do just that. Together we can get clarity on what you want to achieve as parents, and as a couple, and build a solid foundation on which to grow.

HOW TO USE THIS BOOK

This is a workbook, designed for you to scribble and take notes on, and to process and troubleshoot some of the questions I'm going to throw your way. Each section has room for notes so that as you come up with ideas you can easily return to them.

You will want to set aside some time each night to answer a few questions, or tackle one whole section at a time. Go at the pace that works for you. You'll need a pen and possibly a notepad, though ideally there is enough room in the workbook for you to jot down your answers.

This process is about getting you both discussing ideas and plans. Nothing needs to be a firm answer. Let it be a fun activity in preparing you to welcome your little one.

A little note:

I'm well aware that parents and families come in all shapes and sizes. Among my own friendship circle there are families with moms and dads, dads and dads, moms and moms, single parents, adoptive parents, and blended families. To simplify matters for the purpose of this book, I will predominately use the term "mom" for the primary caregiver/stay-at-home parent for the first few months, even though I'm well aware that these days this title and role can be much more fluid.

I have also chosen to predominately use the word "partner" when referring to a second parent or co-parent, though in describing my personal stories I use the words "daddy" or "father" because that is the language we use in our family.

Finally, this book is relationship focused and does assume that there is a partnership in place. However, single parents can still benefit greatly from engaging with many of these questions to ensure they are prepared with the support they will need once they bring their little one home.

A second little note:

You are probably hearing a lot about how hard parenthood it going to be, and I'm sorry to say that my book is no exception. I hope that the work you do within these pages can make parenthood significantly easier and your transition smoother. But I'm not going to lie—parenthood *is* hard.

However, let me also say that it is *magical*. Beyond words magical. It is worth every hard moment when your little person says "I love you" for the first time, or takes his or her first steps, or giggles uncontrollably, or rests that little head on your shoulder. Truly, parenthood is the best thing that will ever happen to you, so please keep that excitement and joy in the back of your mind as you prepare. I promise, it will all be worth it.

Okay! On to section one.

SECTION ONE: FAMILY VALUES

This section is going to ask you questions that are designed to get you thinking about your family values, which will be the foundation and framework for the way you choose to raise your children. These values will be what you return to each time you are unsure of the right answer or the best approach to take. They will also help guide you toward the literature and support that best suits your parenting style, helping you focus on the tools that will truly help you personally as you move into parenthood.

QUESTION #1

Think about your journey to parenthood (was it straightforward, did it take a long time, have you always wanted children, was this pregnancy a surprise, etc.?). How do you think this will impact your experience? Consider both the positive and negative ways it might impact you.

Each partner should answer individually, then discuss together.

Our experiences leading up to having a child can dramatically affect our experience of parenthood. For example, I've often seen women who have struggled to have a baby (and after years of trying finally do) go through deep postpartum depression that is further exacerbated by feeling that they should be "so happy." After all, they worked so hard and waited so long for this.

On the other hand, I've also seen couples who end up with a surprise pregnancy struggle with hard feelings, including resentment, after a baby is born because they hadn't planned for this life change.

On the flip side, a long struggle to have a baby can often create a joy that is unaffected by the challenges of parenthood; both parents are just so happy the baby is finally here that nothing seems to faze them. Or, in the case of the surprise pregnancy, both parents are so taken with their little one that all of the worry and resentment seem to fade away.

There is no way to predict these things, but having a sense of how you might be affected can help you prepare for what may happen after baby is born.

In terms of parenting itself, our personal parenting journeys can greatly impact our parenting choices. For example, couples who have struggled with infertility may find themselves more susceptible to setting looser boundaries with their children because they are so overjoyed with their new family that they want to do anything to make their little ones happy. On the other hand, couples who experience unplanned pregnancies may be more rigid in their parenting style in an attempt to keep aspects of their old life intact.

These are generalizations of course. I've seen couples with all kinds of journeys into parenthood have varying experiences. The point here is to get you thinking about how your own journey may sway your choices one way or another, or how it may impact you emotionally one way or another.

If you think your experience may make you more laid back than you would like to be, you can consider ways in which to offset that if you choose. If you worry that you will be too strict or rigid, you might consider things that will increase relaxation and ease in day-to-day choices.

This conversation is simply a way of getting in touch with some of the possibilities that may arise from your experience so that when and if they occur you are not only prepared for the feelings themselves, you are also prepared for how to handle them.

NOTES ON QUESTION #1

QUESTION #2

What most excites you about becoming a parent?

QUESTION #3

What makes you the most nervous about becoming a parent?

Each partner should answer individually, then discuss together.

It's important to share with one another which aspects of parenthood most excite you personally so that as a team you can work toward enhancing those experiences when they arise. It's equally important to share the things that scare you or worry you as individuals. You may find that these thoughts are similar to one another, or they may be different. Either way, voicing the fears and concerns allows you an opportunity to troubleshoot. Once those fears are out there, take the time to really think about what plans you can put in place to set yourselves up for success.

For example, if you are worried about not getting enough sleep (most people are!) you might want to consider doing shift work overnight. Shift work is where you divide the night into two parts (say, 9 p.m.–2 a.m. and 2 a.m.–7 a.m.) and each of you takes a shift. This way each person is getting a somewhat longer chunk of rest each night AND each person is taking on responsibility overnight, thus lessening the resentment that can build between couples when one partner is up all night and the other is snoring away for eight hours. If mom is nursing, her partner can bring her the baby to nurse on his or her shift, but will then take care of all changing, burping, soothing, and getting baby back to sleep. Shift work is also an amazing way to create bonding between baby and the co-parent because the latter is actively involved in baby's care.

Let's say that you are worried about not getting enough time together as a couple. This is a great opportunity to get a plan in place for date night or "together time." If you have family nearby, ask them *now* how often they might be willing to take the baby for an hour or two so you can spend some baby-free time with your partner. Or, if you don't have extra help at hand, think about ways in which you can prioritize your couple time. My husband and I used to take fifteen minutes every night when our babies were asleep and *start* by snuggling on the couch and checking in about how our day was. We prioritized this over dinner, the dishes, the laundry, etc. because it was our way of making sure we connected each day beyond addressing necessary tasks.

These are just examples of how you might troubleshoot some of the concerns that may come up from question #3. The goal is to voice the concern and then really look at what you can do *now* to plan and prepare for those things should they come up. You'll find it is so much easier to discuss these things now than when baby is here and you are tired and focused on your little one.

NOTES ON QUESTIONS #2 & #3

QUESTION #4

What is your overall goal for your child? Who (or what) do you wish them to be?

It might be helpful to start by choosing a single word (e.g.: successful, happy, smart, beautiful, kind, etc.) to describe how you wish to raise them and which traits you hope they will develop as they grow.

If you find you cannot hone in on a single word, choose instead to focus on a concept or phrase.

I want my child to be _____

How do you each define that concept?

What has that concept looked like for you in the past (this could be your own childhood experience or other life experiences where you have felt this way)?

What steps does a person take to achieve this word or concept?

What choices as a parent do you need to make in order to help your child achieve this word or concept?

This question should be discussed and answered as a couple.

This is a big question, and a key element to this workbook. In order to avoid the "winging it" approach to parenthood we have to create a sense of what we are trying to achieve. At the end of the day, when you bring a child into the world you are choosing to be responsible for how that child contributes to society as a fully formed adult. You are literally in charge of helping to shape their views on the things that matter. So "winging it" doesn't sound like such a good plan when we think of it in this way.

And in order to figure out what we want to achieve—who we wish our little ones to be—we have to ask ourselves what is our one core goal. And that answer will be different for everyone.

Once you have identified a key overarching goal, the next question asks you to define the word or concept you have chosen. What does "happy" or "kind" or "successful" *mean* to you? Again, this will be different for everyone but you might be starting to see how having a goal, and then defining it, will allow you later to get a sense of whether or not you are achieving that goal.

For example, my answer is *happy*. My goal as a mother is to raise children who are truly, deeply happy. I define happiness as the ability to notice and collect happy moments, so that when life throws challenges your way you are buffered by all of the times you have noticed your own happiness. It doesn't make the hard stuff easier, it just allows it to be a part of a bigger picture so it's not the only thing we see. True happiness, to me, is the ability to continue to notice happy things even in the face of adversity, for this is a true and balanced life. To me, then, happiness embodies other words like "grateful" and "loving" because they are connected to the ability to notice one's own happiness.

So, when my son comes bounding down the stairs and says "Mommy I'm so happy right now!" or my daughter declares, "This is the best day ever!" or either one exclaims, "My heart is so full right now!" then I know I'm achieving my goal. They are noticing the happy moments day to day and that will buffer the heartache when it inevitably comes. They have honed this skill, and that was my goal as a mother.

That is a long-winded explanation of these first two steps. And, of course, I want many more things for my kids than just happiness, and there are many more ways for me to know that they are happy, but this helps me hone in on the core, the root of my goal, so that it can be my foundation as a parent moving forward.

Next, ask yourselves what this concept has looked like for you in the past. How have you experienced it? What has it looked like for each of you as individuals? Coming back to my example of happiness, for me it is a warm feeling in my heart. I've learned to spot this feeling clearly; sometimes it is there when I am enjoying coffee with a friend, or on a sunny day in Seattle when Mt. Rainier is visible in all her glory. In these moments, I feel that warmth in my heart and I notice my happiness.

In harder times, when life had thrown serious challenges my way, I still knew I was happy because even through the heartache I had moments of joy that I could feel and notice.

So, if you chose "kind," or "successful," or "smart," or "happy," what has that idea looked like for you in the past?

How do you recognize it? How do you then teach your child to recognize it?

The next step is to look at your own experiences and ask yourselves what does it take to achieve that? How does one become kind, or smart, or successful or happy or . . . ?

And finally, you need to ask yourselves which choices you, as parents, need to make in order to help your children take what was once a concept and turn it into who they are.

Even though my goal is for my children to be happy, I don't think this means they have to be happy all the time. Happiness to me is about noticing that feeling and collecting it so that it doesn't get lost. If I wanted them to be happy every minute of the day, I wouldn't be setting boundaries. And ultimately, when they went into the world, which is full of boundaries, they would be sorely disappointed and grossly unprepared, causing them *unhappiness*, instead. Therefore, *our* steps as parents are to ensure that they are taught how to notice their own happy feelings and are given the boundaries necessary for them to hone the experience of feeling joy even when things aren't exactly as we wish them to be.

NOTES ON QUESTION #4

QUESTION #5

What are your family values?

Write down five to ten core values you wish to impart to your child and define each of these values in a single sentence (see examples at the end of this section). You do not have to have ten, but please do not list more than that:

1.

2.

3.

4.

5.

6.

7.

8.

9.

10.

This prompt should be answered and discussed as a couple. Please note that this question can take some time so you may choose to treat it as a single session.

This question is designed to build a framework in your home that you can rely on as you navigate all the things that parenthood will throw your way. Having a strong sense of your family values will enable you to return to this list anytime you are unsure of how to handle a situation. This list will also help you teach your child these values as you continue to refer back to them along your parenting journey.

Let's imagine that one of the values on your list is tenacity. Here is how my family defines tenacity:

Going after what we want, embracing failure as an opportunity to learn, then trying again.

Here are a few examples of how you might parent to this value as you move along through parenthood:

- Your toddler is learning to take her off her shoes. She gets frustrated easily because her little hands just can't quite master the proper grip. As you watch her struggle, your heart yearns to help her get those shoes off so she doesn't have to suffer anymore. But in your family, you value tenacity. So instead, you choose to sit with her while she learns, encouraging her and praising her *tenacity* as she works hard to learn how to do this. In this moment not only are you, yourself, living and teaching the value but you are also naming it for your child in such a way that it will become a part of her own foundation and vocabulary.

- Your son begged to be on the swim team. Now he hates it because he can't master the crawl stroke. As he begs you to let him quit, you know that your family values tenacity and that you want to impart this value more than you want to make him comfortable. So, when you talk with him about it, you may say something like, "I know it's hard and frustrating when you can't figure something out. Tenacity is important in our family and so you can quit once you have mastered the crawl stroke or once the summer is over, whichever comes first. Learning can feel hard, but every time you get it wrong it's an opportunity to get better. Failure is sometimes how we learn." Here again you are making this tough decision based on your family values. You know that you cannot let him quit without trying to learn and grow and still uphold your foundational values. And so, it makes the decision a little clearer and a little easier when you can both mentally and literally refer back to these family values in this way.

Now, it goes without saying that you may need to tweak these values as you grow into parenthood. And you may feel that valuing tenacity looks different in your family than it does in the examples above (or tenacity might not make your list of Family Values at all). Either way, the previous examples aren't answers, they're just a way of showing you how making these choices now can gently support you on your parenting journey so you aren't simply "winging it."

Family Values Example:

Love: We hope it comes easily and work at it when it doesn't.

Gratitude: We are truly thankful for what we already have and take the time to notice it.

Compassion: We show kindness and concern for others, and seek to understand them.

Integrity: We say and do the right thing even when no one is looking.

Forgiveness: We recognize our own humanity in others.

Tenacity: We go after what we want, embrace failure as an opportunity to learn, then try again.

Creativity: we know when to follow our own path and think outside the box.

Generosity: We give of our time, talent, and wealth to those who need us.

Friendship: We show up for the people we love in good times and bad, and celebrate their successes as if they were our own.

Courage: We know that sometimes fear comes along for the ride, but we never let it sit in the driver's seat.

NOTES ON QUESTION #5

QUESTION #6

What three things do you see other parents doing that you wish to emulate?

1.

2.

3.

Share your thoughts individually, then discuss as a couple.

I love this question because one of the best ways to become a great parent is to watch other great parents and do what they do! I have several friends who are my guides as I navigate parenthood and whom I channel when things get tough. Think about this question in several different ways (you are welcome to come up with more than three things if you like):

- how they engage with their children;

- how they interact with each other as partners; and

- how they care for themselves as individuals.

Each aspect is equally important to experiencing a balanced parenting journey.

NOTES ON QUESTION #6

QUESTION #7

What three things do you see other parents doing that you wish to avoid?

1.

2.

3.

Share your thoughts individually, then discuss as a couple.

On the flip side, one of the best ways to become a great parent is to learn from your friends' mistakes. The truth is you don't really know how to be a great parent until you become a parent, and you will make a million mistakes along the way. It's inevitable. So as your friends make mistakes, learn from them by thinking about how you might like to handle a situation differently. HOWEVER, this is a tricky piece of advice because one of the other crazy things that happens when you become a parent is that you suddenly understand how some of these mistakes happen—and you may even choose to make the same ones.

The difference in this instance is that making these mistakes is a *choice*. I'll give you an example from my own life:

Years before I became a mother myself I bought a birthday gift for a friend's little one. The child was about three or four at the time. One day shortly thereafter I was dropping something off at my friend's house and as we stood at the door she called out to her child to come and say thank you for the gift. The child refused. My friend pushed again. Again, the child refused. And so, my friend turned to me and said, "They say thank you for the gift."

At the time I was appalled. I literally came home and relayed the story to my husband declaring I would NEVER let our future, unborn child do something like that. We would return the gift if they couldn't show gratitude.

Flash forward a few years and suddenly I have twin three-year-olds. An almost identical situation happens. In my head I remembered this incident with my friend and my heartfelt declaration. But in my heart, this just wasn't a battle I wanted to fight publicly. I was exhausted; three is a lot younger than I had realized, and honestly this was a chance to have a conversation about gratitude, not force a meaningless "thank you" out of our children.

And so, I did what I swore I would never do and said, "They loved your gift. We are going to have a little chat later about how important it is to show gratitude. Thank you so much for giving it to them." When I talked with my kids later on, we decided to follow up with a thank you drawing that we mailed to my friend the next day.

While having a sense of what we don't want to do as parents is important, I would argue that knowing what you *do* want is a far better plan. I knew in that moment that my goal was to impart a sense of gratitude, and that a forced "thank you" at the door wasn't how we would accomplish that goal.

Try to look at the mistakes your friends make as ways of helping you determine what you *do* want—and use a loving eye, because soon you will be the one in the hot seat, and believe me you are going to make mistakes that others can learn from, too!

NOTES ON QUESTION #7

QUESTION #8

Do you know about the various parenting choices/styles out there and, if so, are you leaning toward one of them? (e.g.: attachment parenting, sleep training, scheduled feeding, co-sleeping, etc.)

Share your thoughts individually, then discuss as a couple.

One of the best ways to avoid the "winging it" type of parenting is to get a sense of what philosophies are out there that may resonate with you. Once you find the one that meets your core values and sounds the most likely to help you achieve the parenting experience and the home environment that works for your family, you can then focus your time reading the specific literature that resonates with you.

Of course, you can change your mind once baby arrives, but oftentimes a particular philosophy resonates with a couple's core values, and identifying that philosophy can lead you to further guidance through literature, blogs, etc. Below you will find just a few of the choices, philosophies, and resources available. Please note that more than one style of parenting may resonate with you! Feel free to cherry pick, so to speak. All of the concepts are there to help you build up your personal parenting approach and framework for raising your little one.

Gentle Sleep Training:
Suzy Giordano, *The Baby Sleep Solution*

Marc Weissbluth, M.D., *Healthy Sleep Habits, Happy Child*

Kim West and Joanne Kenen, *The Sleep Lady's Good Night, Sleep Tight: Gentle Proven Solutions to Help Your Child Sleep Well and Wake Up Happy*

Sleep training is best defined as teaching your child how to sleep through the night. There are various styles which lean all the way from letting babies "cry it out" to gently encouraging and habituating them to fall asleep without you present and then stay asleep throughout the night.

There are mixed views out there about this technique. Many parents who have used it swear by it (myself included) but there are concerns that long periods of crying can interfere with baby's attachment and feelings of security.

Sleep training can be especially useful for parents who don't do well on very little sleep, parents of multiples, or parents who are more schedule oriented, as oftentimes sleep training requires a solid bedtime (and sometimes daytime) schedule.

Attachment Parenting:

William Sears and Martha Sears, *The Attachment Parenting Book: A Commonsense Guide to Understanding and Nurturing Your Baby*

William Sears, Martha Sears, Robert Sears, and James Sears, *The Baby Book*

William Sears, Martha Sears, Robert Sears, and James Sears, *The Baby Sleep Book*

Attachment parenting swings the other way and focuses on building attachment between a baby and its parents. This approach often encourages on-demand feeding (as opposed to sleep training, which may lean more toward scheduled feeding), co-sleeping, and a quick responsiveness from parents in order for baby to feel secure.

Attachment parenting may raise some concerns when it comes to parents getting their own sleep needs met (whether it's getting enough sleep or physically having space in bed at night), as well as having day-to-day independence from their little one. There are also risks associated with co-sleeping and SIDS, though you do not need to co-sleep in order to practice attachment parenting.

Attachment parenting is well suited to parents who are less schedule oriented and still function well on limited sleep. It can also be something that parents feel most comfortable practicing if their own parents did not provide secure attachment for them.

Fostering Emotional Intelligence in Children (for children age 12 months+):

John Gottman, *Raising an Emotionally Intelligent Child*

Foster Cline and Jim Fay, *Love and Logic*

Jane Nelson, *Positive Discipline*

Parents who wish to develop emotionally intelligent children focus on helping children understand, as well as name, their feelings in order to lessen tantrums and create more happy, mentally healthy children and future adults.

Raising children with emotional intelligence can also help them have stronger interpersonal relationships and a greater empathy for others. I can tell you that as a parent coach and mental health professional this is a huge focal point of the work I do, so I'm a huge fan of this philosophy.

Choosing the right philosophy for you:

Now that you have a sense of some of the various styles of parenting in our modern world, give some thought to who you are as a couple and as individuals. Do any of these styles resonate? It may be that more than one feels right to you and that's ok, too! Most parents don't follow one style in its entirety, but oftentimes take the parts they like from each and run with those. And really, these styles and choices are just a few—there are plenty more out there to choose from!

The key is that the style matches who you are as a person. If you are schedule oriented, on-demand feeding might feel challenging to you. If you are more relaxed and go with the flow, you may not feel comfortable sticking with the routine required for sleep training.

What matters most is that you are happy and content as a parent, so that you can truly show up for your little one. Where I'm always concerned is when someone feels pressured by family, a peer group, or society in general to pick a style that they are told is "best for baby" and which leaves them feeling wrecked or floundering.

What's best for your baby is that you feel confident, happy, and healthy. Start there and the rest will follow.

NOTES ON QUESTION #8

QUESTION #9

Finally, what was the best parenting choice your parent(s) made for you when you were growing up? Which was the worst?

Share your thoughts individually, then discuss as a couple.

Here is where you each get to look at your own childhood experience and ask yourself (as you may already have done) what you would like to do the same. What would you like to do the differently? Even people with the best childhood experiences usually still find a few things they would like to do differently with their own children.

And if you had the kind of childhood where your parent(s) did nothing right by you, then you have a chance to wipe the slate clean and start fresh, to take all those things that you wish had been different and make them different for *your* little one.

Finally, after you've had a chance to look at the influence your parents had and what you might repeat vs. what you might do differently, take a moment to remember that each child is unique and it is important to parent them in the way *they* need to be parented. While it is extremely important that we learn from our own parents' mistakes and successes, it can also be detrimental to be hard set about any of it. Your child is not you, and therefore you may find that it is necessary to repeat what felt like a "mistake" for you in the interest of your own child's needs. And parenthood has a wonderful way of helping us understand our parents just that little bit more, and shed light on the choices they made in a whole new way. The bottom line? Be prepared to be flexible!

NOTES ON QUESTION #9

SECTION TWO:
THE FIRST FEW MONTHS

Before we dive into the next set of questions I want you to do a little exercise. First, I want you to jot down on the lines below all of the things you think are going to change or need to be redefined once your baby arrives. Things like cooking, cleaning, exercise, and sleep, come to mind. Think of as many as you can and together make a nice long list.

I have provided a list on the next page as oftentimes there are things couples don't think of right off the bat, but please don't skip to that list. I encourage you to start by making your own list before you look at mine. Trust me, this will be more helpful in the long run.

THINGS THAT WILL NEED TO BE RETHOUGHT OR REDEFINED ONCE BABY ARRIVES:

_____ _____ _____
_____ _____ _____
_____ _____ _____
_____ _____ _____
_____ _____ _____
_____ _____ _____
_____ _____ _____
_____ _____ _____

Now that you've made your list, compare it to my list below and add anything you were missing:

Sleep
Showering
Doing hair
Doing makeup
Brushing teeth
Going to the bathroom (yes, I mean peeing and pooping need to be redefined)
Cooking
Eating
Cleaning the house
Dishes
Laundry
Grocery Shopping
Exercise
Sex
Date nights
Me time
Work/life balance
Pets
Travel
Money
Reading
Time with friends

It's a little scary right? I know. But here's the thing: seeing it on paper like this is important because now you won't be quite so surprised when you realize you haven't brushed your teeth one day. You are planning for it.

Now I want you to use the worksheet in the pages that follow to organize these things into three categories. You should do this individually because each of you will have different priorities.

Things I Will Prioritize

In the "things I will prioritize" category start by naming your top five things you would want to prioritize each day.

Then, narrow those five down to a total of thirty minutes. As in, the new list should collectively take no more than thirty minutes combined. If you have something that takes twenty minutes, you may have to go down to just two or three things on this list.

These are the things that you absolutely MUST prioritize every day, the things that make you feel like a human being, and on which you and your partner will work together to ensure they get met each and every day. This list might change once your baby is born, but let's at least start this conversation now. For me, shower was at the top of this list. I could go without brushing my teeth but heaven forbid I skipped a shower!

It's important to literally prioritize these (as in the most important thing each day, the second most important thing each day, etc.) so that when you catch a moment for yourself you know exactly what to do first!

People can get frustrated when making this list, especially if something on it takes thirty minutes in and of itself—then what? The thing is, there will be lots of days where you get more than thirty minutes to yourself, and then you can tackle those other things. But on the days when time is tight, and parenthood seems to be taking up every moment of your day, I want to make sure that your most basic needs are being met and that you are able to prioritize them, instead of frittering those precious minutes away on something that isn't as important as your basic needs.

I was working with a couple recently and the co-parent said, "I just don't understand why I need to put going to the bathroom on here. I mean, if I have to go to the bathroom I'll just go." I smiled remembering the times that I really needed to go to the bathroom and I couldn't because I had a crying baby who was covered in poop, or pee, or puke, and that cleanup had to be prioritized over my needs.

And even though right now your mind probably can't quite comprehend how you might have to prioritize going to the bathroom, this book is all about what you don't know yet. So please, do the exercise, even if you think I'm crazy. You just might thank me for it later.

Things I Can Ask for Help With

In the "things I can ask for help with" category put all of the things that someone else *could* do for you. Things like cooking, cleaning, and folding laundry go on this list.

Things I Will Let Go of For Now

And finally, in the "things I will let go of for now" list put everything else. This just might be your longest list.

Parent One:

Things I Will Prioritize	Things I Can Ask for Help With	Things I Will Let Go of For Now

Parent Two:

Things I Will Prioritize	Things I Can Ask for Help With	Things I Will Let Go of For Now

How to use these lists:

The "things I will prioritize" list should be shared with your partner and any other individual who will be involved in the first weeks of baby's life. Once you have shared what your priorities are, it becomes easier to figure out a plan to make those things happen. For example, my priority was a shower. For me, showering is how I feel like I am ready to face the world. So, my husband and I worked out that he would get up for work fifteen minutes early each day so that I could have my shower.

My husband, on the other hand, needed some down time to transition between work and home. His priority was having ten minutes alone (ideally with a beer in hand) before he was on "daddy duty."

Now, imagine if we hadn't planned for this. My husband, not knowing that he was my only hope of snagging a shower each day, would have gotten up to go to work at his normal time, and likely would have returned home, grabbed a beer, and taken ten minutes for himself. Recipe for disaster? I think so.

If we don't have these conversations then we don't know how to support each other and make sure that our basic needs are getting met each day. It sounds silly but simply getting your basic needs met not only helps you feel more "normal" as you transition into parenthood, but it also makes you feel like you are being cared for by your partner.

These priorities might change once your baby is born. You may discover that you can live without a shower but you really need twenty minutes on the treadmill every morning, and that's ok! Because it sure is easier to make that change once the conversation has already happened than it is to try and begin the conversation with a crying baby in your arms when you are both functioning on only a few hours of sleep. Discuss it now and make it that much easier on the other side to get those needs met.

The "things I can ask for help with" list should be hung on your fridge. Once baby arrives it is normal for friends and family to come and visit and say kind things like "what can I do to help?" It's equally normal for parents to feel so overwhelmed that they honestly can't think of a single thing when put on the spot, despite being surrounded by laundry and dirty dishes. Having a list on the fridge allows you to say, "there's a list on the fridge––pick anything! We are so grateful!" This empowers your friends and family to actually help you without you having to do the hard work of figuring out what you need in that moment. It also allows people to pick a task they are comfortable with, instead of being asked to take out your trash, when they might really, really hate taking out the trash, but secretly love folding the laundry.

The final and, perhaps, most important list is "things I will let go of." This list is all about setting realistic expectations for yourselves as new parents. This list is probably long and includes really tough stuff like me time, time with friends, travel, and a host of other things you have no intention of giving up. But here is the truth: for now, you may have to. **And here is the bigger truth: if you make peace with this idea—that it's just *for now*—you will open the door to feeling like a balanced and accomplished person as you transition into parenthood.**

Look at all the stuff on your lists! You are probably barely getting those things done now and you don't yet have a newborn. Readjusting your expectations about what you can achieve each day is the key to feeling like you are achieving things.

Think of it this way: if you are thinking you can have a newborn, keep the house clean, do your hair and makeup each day, hit the gym, and still have dinner on the table by 7:00 p.m. then how will you feel on a day where none of that gets done? Probably a bit like a failure. Whereas if you say "OK, my goal today is to shower, brush my teeth, and sit down to eat breakfast," then imagine how you'll feel if you do get a workout in *and* manage to fold a load of laundry. You'll feel like a superhero! And let me tell you, every day you keep your baby fed and healthy you are, quite literally, a superhero.

So, readjust those expectations for a short while. You'll be amazed how many things come back to you in just a few months' time. In fact, I encourage couples to pull out this last list on baby's first birthday and check off all the things that have already returned to normal (or the things it turns out you no longer care about returning to normal).

Now for those of you like me, who define themselves as organized planners, and think you will literally turn into a slovenly beast should you lower your expectations by even 20 percent —do it anyway. Put a boundary around it if you like ("this is only for the first three months"), but please, I beg of you, do it. Because this list is the most important one I didn't make, and if I had, I truly believe I would have had a much gentler transition into parenthood. I would have realized that I was, quite frankly, a superhero by keeping two babies fed, changed, and happy. And the rest of that stuff, well, it just wasn't as important as I thought it was.

The First Few Months Questions:

QUESTION #1

What will each person's role be overnight? More specifically, what is the co-parent's job going to be overnight? If the plan is for your partner to sleep, how will they contribute in the mornings and evenings before bed? Will they participate differently on the weekends? If the plan is to work as a team, you might consider the shift work discussed in section one.

Share your thoughts individually, then discuss as a couple.

Here's the deal: when you bring a new baby home the only person who should be well rested is the baby. Period. You are a team, and trust me, teamwork doesn't stop just because one person has breasts with milk in them and the other doesn't. Everyone should be participating overnight.

Even if one of you has to "go to work" in the morning, the truth is you *both* have hard work to do in the morning, so there is no reason you can't both be involved overnight. And yes, OK, one of you has the goods (as in the breasts with milk) but there is a lot more to the work overnight than just feeding. Burping, changing, soothing, washing up pumping equipment, searching for lost pacifiers—these are all things that either partner can do.

So please, discuss this. Talk about how each person is going to be involved. Without a feeling of teamwork all sorts of issues arise. Most often, this is where a general resentment can build up between a couple. If mom is up all night while her partner snores for eight hours, she begins to feel that she is all alone. This can cause depression, anger, frustration, and many more hard feelings, so many of which can be avoided by her partner being just that: a partner.

But some other interesting things come up when one partner is absent overnight. Namely, that partner tends to not have the same ability to meet their baby's needs and baby begins to want mom only. Babies change so quickly, sometimes day to day, and often what worked to soothe the baby on Monday might not work come Thursday. If one parent has been out of the house all day, and then isn't up at night participating, that parent might try to use that trick from Monday, when mom knows it doesn't work anymore. She'll begin to get frustrated. Eventually she'll say, "give me the baby" and take over for her partner .

In that moment two important things happen: First, mom feels like she does everything because her partner doesn't even know how to soothe the baby. Second, her partner feels powerless, as though mom doesn't trust them to do anything. And from here tension and hard feelings can arise.

So, do yourselves a favor and function as a true team. It will only serve to make you stronger, better parents and a far better couple (even if one of you is a bit more sleep deprived than you may have originally anticipated).

NOTES ON QUESTION #1

QUESTION #2

Thinking back to the earlier list of "things I will prioritize," which of those priority needs are you most worried about continuing to meet once baby is born? How can your partner help you meet that need?

Share your thoughts individually, then discuss as a couple.

This question is so important to troubleshoot with your partner. If you each know which thing is most important on your list, or which one you are most worried you might lose, your partner can work hard to keep an eye on it and prioritize it with you. I say "with you" because **you have to prioritize it, too**. Parenthood can easily turn into martyrdom if you aren't careful, so make sure you are committed to prioritizing your own needs as well as your baby's.

It becomes as simple as ensuring your partner gets this need met every day. "Honey, have you had your shower yet today?" or "Now would be a great time for you to go for your run" are a few ways of carving out the time your partner's needs, but more importantly it's a message of love and support. It is a way of saying "I see you, I love you, I want to care for you."

NOTES ON QUESTION #2

QUESTION #3

Which of your *partner's* priority needs are you most worried about continuing to meet once baby is born? How can we troubleshoot that worry *now*?

Share your thoughts individually, then discuss as a couple.

Looking at those three lists and focusing on the "things I will prioritize" list, think about which of your partner's priorities *you* are most worried about being able to help them prioritize. This doesn't have to be a cause for anger or frustration on anyone's part, just an opportunity to say "That might be hard. Let's talk about how we achieve that." It's important to think about which priorities might be hard to fulfill because having them unmet can easily be misinterpreted as you not caring for your partner's needs. However, if you discuss this subject beforehand, it's a lot easier to be forgiving.

NOTES ON QUESTION #3

QUESTION #4

What is your plan for communicating/troubleshooting in the first few months of parenthood?

Discuss as a couple.

Like it or not, you will bump heads in the first months of bringing baby home. Lack of sleep can turn even the best communicators into their worst selves, so it's best to be prepared. I worked with a couple who decided, "We should just forget everything we said to each other in the first year after our son was born. It just shouldn't count! We didn't mean any of it!"

So, think about how you communicate at your worst, and how you argue at your worst, and then discuss what issues you think may arise from being in this unique time and how you might avoid or resolve them. And digging even further, think about what issues between the two of you might get triggered by sleep deprivation and a lot of task-oriented work. Is there a history of one partner doing more than the other? That could come up at 3:00 a.m.!

Discuss how you can troubleshoot at 3:00 a.m. Maybe you decide to always discuss things in the morning, or maybe you think about which ways of communicating in the past have been most helpful for each of you and which ways could be most detrimental.

NOTES ON QUESTION #4

QUESTION #5

How is maternity/paternity leave going to work and what feelings does each of you have surrounding this topic?

Share your thoughts individually, then discuss as a couple.

Chances are you have already discussed this topic, perhaps in great detail. I bring it up less as an opportunity to problem solve and more as an opportunity to share whatever feelings this unique time brings up for you. Is either one of you resentful that one of you will be home? Is either one of you seeing this as a "break" for the person taking time off? Are there any disagreements about how much time off the non-stay-at-home parent will be taking?

There is a common misconception that the person taking leave is about to go on a short vacation. In fact, I always inwardly giggle when moms in my childbirth education class say how much they are looking forward to some "time off work." Let me be the first to squash any beliefs you may have that this is "time off." In fact, I would argue that the person staying home is often working the hardest, because they have to do it without hot coffee, a hot meal (sometimes without any lunch at all), and is at the beck and call of the most demanding boss they've ever had, all without feeling like they've actually achieved anything or successfully solved any problems all day long. So, let's just put that idea to the side, shall we?

Coming at this with the awareness that whoever is staying home for those first months is hard at work, too, will help the two of you come together each evening to share your personal experiences of working hard, instead of one seeing the other's work as "time off."

This happens in reverse, too, by the way. Parents stuck at home with a crying baby can easily yearn for the trials and tribulations of that office job they had before the baby was born, forgetting what it's like to try and do all of that on only a few hours of sleep while missing their little ones and knowing that they only get to see them for a few hours each day.

NOTES ON QUESTION #5

QUESTION #6

How will you prioritize and care for your relationship *as a couple* in the first few months of parenthood? Which key activities in your relationship do both of you want to preserve during your transition into parenthood? Be realistic here, as you aren't going to be able to preserve everything, so focus on one or two things that you feel really connect you.

Share your thoughts individually, then discuss as a couple.

This question is incredibly important as all too often couples become task-oriented after a baby is born and lose the connection they had when they created this little person in the first place.

Finding that connection can be as simple as putting aside fifteen minutes each day to connect and talk or as complex as finding a sitter for a weekly date night. Whatever it is, in whatever way you do it, planning for couple time is essential to feeling connected through the transition into parenthood.

Task-oriented achievements are great, and will definitely create a sense of teamwork, but beyond being a great team, you need to maintain a great connection and deep love for one another.

In our house we used something called "Rose and Thorn." I believe we stole this from the Obamas but don't quote me on that. Each night we would sit down for fifteen minutes *before* we made dinner, did the dishes, or tidied up, and we would share the rose of our day (the best part) and the thorn of our day (the hardest part).

Oftentimes I would get far more information from my husband about his day this way than I did when I said, "How was your day?" and he replied with, "Fine." When we played "Rose and Thorn" I'd hear about the big meeting that went well or the project that went south. And he would hear more details about the funny things our kiddos did that day or the stuff that made me want to pull my hair out. It truly gave us a better sense of what actually happened that day in just a short period of time.

Flash forward to the present day and our kids now participate in this game over the dinner table each night. They love it and we love it because, once again, we find out a lot more about their day this way.

And to boot, this exercise links to our overarching goal of raising happy children, because every day we encourage them to find the joy by searching for that rose, while still acknowledging that it's normal for life to have thorns along the way.

So give some thought to how you will carve out connection time each day together. Will it be "Rose and Thorn?" Watching a favorite show each night? Playing your favorite board game? Listening to a podcast? How will you truly connect when time is tight and energy is low?

NOTES ON QUESTION #6

QUESTION #7

Does Mom intend to breastfeed? If so, how important to you is this choice on a scale of one to ten, ten being "I will be devastated if I cannot breastfeed"? How will you work as partners to achieve your breastfeeding goal? Finally, which (if any) scenarios would make you decide to stop trying?

The birthing mother should share her thoughts, and then you should discuss as a couple.

I ask this question only to have you think about what it might be like if breastfeeding is a struggle, or if you simply can't do it. I see time and time again women who so deeply wanted to breastfeed feel absolutely sideswiped when they can't or when they struggle for one reason or another.

If you put down a ten for this answer, then of course you must persevere! I ask this question so that you begin to engage with the feelings that may arise if things don't go according to plan, and also to talk about what your partner's role will be in supporting the breastfeeding experience. How might they be able to help, even if you're the one breastfeeding? Could they be in charge of keeping the nursing station stocked, calling around to find a lactation consultant who might be able to help, bring a water bottle while you nurse, or even rub your feet?

Too often partners feel helpless when breastfeeding is a struggle, but they can truly be a part of the solution by taking over any of the additional burdens where no breasts are required! Even something as simple as rubbing mom's feet can send that message that she is loved, that she is doing a great job, and that she is *not alone*.

And finally, I ask you to consider if there are any scenarios that might make you decide to stop trying. For some of you, there aren't any, and that's OK, too.

NOTES ON QUESTION #7

QUESTION #8

Do you have a family history of depression or postpartum depression? Are you worried about this topic? Even if you aren't, do you have a plan for this scenario should it happen to you? Are you aware of how to spot it?

Share your thoughts individually, then discuss as a couple.

I don't want to scare you, but the statistics on women who struggle with some kind of postpartum mood disorder (anxiety, depression, etc.) are really high— something along the lines of three or four in ten. And that's only the women who actually receive a diagnosis. Many more slip through the cracks. And men aren't immune either. Something like one in eighty-four men struggle with a postpartum mood disorder as well. Most expectant parents are thinking about this topic, but most also think it won't happen to them. So, when it does, it can be another version of a sucker punch.

There are some risk factors that you should be aware of, including:

- having a mother who experienced postpartum anxiety or depression;
- having a personal a history of anxiety or depression;
- having more than one baby (twins, triplets, etc.);
- having a baby that was/is in the NICU; and
- having a history of pregnancy loss.

But I also think that women like me, who like to plan, to feel in control, and are career oriented, are more prone to struggling because they are so used to feeling in control of their lives.

If you are at all concerned about this issue, I strongly suggest finding a good therapist now. This way, if you do find yourself struggling, you will know exactly who to call. And, hopefully, you will have had a prenatal session or two so that some rapport has already been built and you aren't starting from scratch. You lose nothing by setting up this relationship now. It will only serve you well to know that it is there should you need it. And a prenatal session or two can be a good way to sort through some of the fears or concerns you may have around this topic.

Professional help aside, it is also worth thinking about how you are going to check in on each other so that any mental health issues can be caught as soon as possible. Having a baby can be a very task-oriented experience and it can be easy to blow off signs of struggle with excuses like "she's tired" or "I didn't eat much today" or "I just need a good night's sleep." While all of that may be true, postpartum struggles go beyond those things and can often impact your view of the world or of your situation.

I say to couples all the time, "you know your partner best. You know her on her best day, her worst day, and how she views the world. You know how she faces a challenge." It is through these considerations that we can begin to notice changes that may go beyond sleep deprivation.

I'll give you a personal example. I'm the kind of person who truly loves the little things in life. A hot cup of coffee, or the sound of my kids giggling, which literally fills my heart with warmth and makes me feel joy in a noticeable way. The area we lived in when my twins were born was covered with trees and our home was at the top of a big hill. Before they were born I would often drive up that hill and the light would stream through the trees in such a way that my heart felt full and I was noticeably happy.

When my children were six weeks old I was driving us all up the hill and the light hit the trees the way it always did, and I realized that I felt nothing. That's when I knew something was wrong. A week later I was diagnosed with postpartum depression (something I had been blowing off with the same excuses listed above and which my husband didn't know how to prod further because, let's be honest, this topic is really *hard*).

So, give some thought as to how either of you might be able to broach this topic if you are concerned. Have a plan for what might be said, so that if you do need to say it, the words themselves aren't new. One couple I worked with had a brilliant system. They called it the "stoplight check-in." Every day they would check in with each other and give their day a color rating (red meaning terrible, yellow meaning just OK, and green meaning good). Over the course of a few days or weeks a pattern might start to emerge. If one partner is reporting mostly reds and yellows, it might be worth having that discussion.

For more information on postpartum mood disorders and how to spot them visit **www.postpartumstress.com**.

NOTES ON QUESTION #8

NOTES

SECTION THREE:
ALL THE MONTHS THEREAFTER

A brief note before I begin: Please don't skip this section. I know these topics seem far away, and you may feel an inclination to put these discussions off until later down the road, but trust me, it is far more challenging to have them later on. Take the time to explore them now and then you can (and will) be able to revisit them later as needed with a foundation of thought already in place.

Now that you've discussed some of your basic needs and organized your priorities for those first few months, let's spend some time figuring out how you can work best as a parenting team when times get tough, as well as how you will prioritize your family time moving forward.

QUESTION #1

How will you carve out time and space for "family time"?

Share your thoughts individually (based on work schedules and home duties), then discuss as a couple.

Spend some time talking not just about what family time means to you, but also how and when family time and work may collide and how you will handle that.

All couples want work/life balance, but not enough spend time thinking about what that actually looks like day to day and planning for how and when focused family time will occur.

Let's say both of you are working but you work different schedules. That's great for childcare, but not so great for family time. Talk about which times/days will be focused on being together. Doing this means that later down the road when there is someone's birthday party on your family day, you'll feel comfortable saying no because you know that this time is set aside for all of you to be together.

Or let's say one of you always works on Saturdays. Perhaps you set Sundays aside for family time so that each week there is quality time together.

If one of you is a stay-at-home parent and the other works, it's equally important to talk about when you are going to be a family, when there are two parents in charge, so that the stay-at-home parent gets a break from their day-to-day role of being the sole caregiver (much like the working parent is getting a break from their work on their days off).

NOTES ON QUESTION #1

QUESTION #2

What will sick days look like when *you* are sick? What will they look like when your child is sick? Think in terms of who stays home, who takes baby to the doctor, how is a healthy baby cared for if either partner is sick, how the stay-at-home partner (if applicable) is cared for if they are sick but baby is healthy, etc.

Discuss as a couple.

I will tell you from my own experience that this was one of the things my husband and I fought about the most. In fact, we didn't actually ask ourselves this question and set an official plan until our twins were five years old. And only then, once I actually agreed to the plan, did the resentment and frustration dissipate, because it was something I *agreed* to.

You see, sick days are something special when it comes to the hardship of parenthood. Sick days are rough, especially if both parents work. Because someone has to stay home. And that someone is usually Mom. And sometimes Mom just can't stay home, and neither can her partner, and so there we are.

Time and time again when my kids were sick I would cancel my clients and feel angry that my work was so much more undervalued in our family than my husband's. I was angry at the world that the expectation was that Mom would stay home. I was angry with my husband's company that it was seen as odd for him to stay home and that this oddity could affect bigger things like bonuses and promotions. *My work matters, too!* I wanted to scream. And one day the worst happened: one of my kids was sick on a work day I *could not miss* and my husband *could not miss* either. It was this minor catastrophe that forced our hands and from which our sick day plan was born.

Taking the time to think about sick days now will prevent a similar catastrophe from happening to you. Knowing what that worst-case scenario plan is will allow you to simply put that plan into motion instead of fighting about it with a sick little one in your arms.

But don't just think about when baby is sick. What about when one of you is sick? Picture this: Mom stays home and her partner works. One day her partner gets sick and stays home. Her partner misses a day of work, lies in bed and sleeps all day (as we do when we are sick). Three days later Mom gets the same bug, but she stays home and cares for baby, so she can't sleep all day to get well. Now mom is not only sick, but she's not set up to get better. And she may be resentful that her partner got a full day of rest and she didn't. Life feels unbalanced and unfair, made worse by the fact that she feels physically awful.

Here is where a plan can really serve you. Maybe the plan is that when Mom gets sick, her partner will always shoulder the load in the morning before work, aim to get home one hour early, and take over as soon as they walk through the door, allowing Mom to head to bed and rest. Maybe the plan is that her partner works from home on sick days. If the partner simply cannot miss work in any way, perhaps there is a neighbor or friend that Mom can call on in times like these. If so, the couple must be sure to talk with them about it now, and not in the midst of a crisis.

The point is, there are usually options, and by having this conversation now you won't have any major surprises later down the line. Instead, you will be dealing with a situation that you had planned for.

NOTES ON QUESTION #2

QUESTION #3

How do you intend to discipline your child?

Share your thoughts individually, then discuss as a couple.

This question is incredibly important because having a framework around discipline will help you feel more prepared when your child surprises you with a moment where discipline is needed.

There are so many schools of thought around this subject and most couples come in with similar views about how to discipline their child, but their views may vary enough to cause confusion if there isn't a clear plan in place.

A great way to break this down is to think first and foremost about what you want your children to *learn* as you discipline them. Do you want to teach them who's in charge? Do you want to help them learn from their mistakes? Is it important to you that children obey? All of these questions will begin to determine the path you take around discipline.

A lot of modern parents are leaning toward the concept of natural consequences, the idea that children should experience the natural consequences of their actions. The book *Love and Logic* is a great example of this style.

Life itself doles out natural consequences to adults (if I don't pay my electric bill, I get my electricity cut off. If I'm late to work too often, I get fired). Helping children understand this from an early age can prevent larger life consequences later down the road.

The natural consequence will vary from situation to situation so it will require some creative thinking on your part, but I'm personally a big fan of this style.

However, many parents want to have a stronger hand and they lean toward sending children to their room, grounding them, or taking privileges away. Again, there isn't a right or wrong, only what is right or wrong for your family (however, it goes without saying that violence toward anyone is never acceptable).

Let's look at a few examples and you can discuss together how you might handle each situation:

Example #1

Your five year old, who is generally a great kid, a good listener, and who is respectful of their things has holes in their comforter. When you ask how this happened they say, "I wanted to see what would happen if I tried to cut it. It made holes!"

How would you handle this situation?

Example #2

Your receive a call from your child's school letting you know that they have been sent to the principal's office for fighting. When you arrive you learn that your child was defending themselves against a bully.

How would you handle this situation?

Example #3

Your three-year-old throws a tantrum to end all tantrums in the grocery store and in the midst of throwing down knocks over a display. (*My child,* you ask? Yup, *your child*).

How would you handle this situation?

Example #4

You bought your child a new bike for their birthday. They were careless and left the bike in the road where a car accidently smashed it.

How would you handle this situation?

All of these scenarios offer teachable moments that call for you as a parent to help your child understand the impact of their actions, but some of them are also public scenarios which may test your own feelings around parenting in an exposed and vulnerable way.

There isn't a right or wrong way to deal with any of these situations, so long as you view them as opportunities to help your child learn and grow. Getting on the same page about how you will do this is key to presenting a strong, united front for your little one, which leads me to the next question.

NOTES ON QUESTION #3

QUESTION #4

How will you provide a united front as parents when you disagree about how to handle a situation?

Discuss as a couple.

I'm sure you are both on the same page about a lot of things, but you will hit points in parenthood where you disagree about how to handle a situation. In fact, you may share the same core value but disagree about how to meet that value, and this may have already come up in the last exercise.

Coming up with a plan for how to make sure both of your points of view are heard and how to work toward a compromise will help you navigate these moments in a calmer and less panicked manner.

Here's a great example: I once worked with a couple who had completely different views on discipline. One thought discipline should be strictly enforced, the other felt incapable of following through with it. But the trickiest part was that the parent who wanted strong discipline left all of the parenting up to the parent who was incapable of enforcing it. As you can imagine, this was a recipe for disaster. Their child didn't get the discipline she needed, and the parents argued all the time because the one who was in charge felt they couldn't do what the other parent felt was important. Now you and I can look at this example objectively and see that perhaps the parent who wanted strong discipline should have taken over where discipline was concerned, if that was something both parents agreed was needed.

But what if you don't agree? When my daughter was five and able to swim I took her to a barbeque party on a lake. My husband couldn't join us but he insisted that I put our daughter in a life vest. I didn't think she needed one but he felt she did. We were discussing this in front of her and eventually it became clear that we weren't going to agree right in this moment.

Our plan for when we disagree has always been to discuss the matter first in front of the children so they can watch us problem solve. Should the discussion ever escalate or reach a point where we might confuse them, we would take the conversation to a separate room and resolve the matter privately. We always prefer that our kids see us figure "it" out, but if we can't right away, we still want them to see us as a united front and know that even when we disagree, we can work together to figure things out as a team.

As we bumped heads and ultimately began to get frustrated with each other, off to our bedroom we went to discuss the life vest matter further. Ultimately, my husband said that when it comes to safety issues, we should always go with the parent who has the greater worry, so that everyone can feel at ease. I agreed that this was fair, and I made sure our daughter wore a life vest at the barbeque. Because we had a plan for how we discuss these things, we were able to solve the problem in five minutes, without it escalating and, most importantly, without our children receiving mixed messages.

Coming across as a united front makes your child feel safer and more secure. It is also a great way to avoid the classic behavior of a child asking one parent for something and getting a "no" then asking the other parent and getting a "yes."

And finally, once you create a united front, remember that if one of you doles out a consequence, the other has to go along for the ride. This means thinking clearly before yelling, "That's it, no TV for the whole day!" as you head out the door to work, leaving the co-parent home to enforce this rule. It also means that should something like this happen, the co-parent must enforce it. Doing your best to work as a team on the front end will help you avoid situations like this one!

So perhaps your plan will be like ours, to step away and try to dig deeper to find out why each person wants to handle a situation the way they want. Or maybe your plan will be to always go with the parent who is predominately in charge because that person will usually have to implement any decision you make. There is no right or wrong here, just your own personal plan for what to do when you disagree; that way, you feel empowered as a team to resolve a situation, instead of feeling lost or resentful when you can't.

NOTES ON QUESTION #4

QUESTION #5

How will you answer the big questions (faith/sex/death/gender/race/etc.)? How will or won't religion play a role in your family? How will you handle your own parents' opinions on how you "should" be imparting values/religion/faith?

Share your thoughts individually, then discuss as a couple.

For some of you this will be an easy answer, but for others it is far more complex. Let's take faith as an example.

My family is mixed faith, made ever more complicated by the fact that my father lives with us. Between the three adults in our home we have a Christian, an atheist, and an agnostic Jew.

Add to that my mother's passing when my children were four and you have a recipe for a lot of big questions with varying answers within one home.

If this is you, you'll want to talk about how you might discuss loss should it arise (and it is likely to at some point, even if it's the loss of a family pet or a friend of the family), as well as how you plan to discuss religion and faith in general in your home. Will you expose your children to the religion you were brought up with? If so, in what ways? How will holidays be acknowledged or celebrated? Will you expose your children to other faiths, or the absence of belief in a higher being?

And don't forget to discuss how your own parents will feel about the choices you are making and how you might choose to handle *that*. This leads us to our next question.

NOTES ON QUESTION #5

QUESTION #6

How will you handle other family members' opinions on the choices you are making?

Share your thoughts individually, then discuss as a couple.

Wouldn't it be great if your parents could remember how hard it was to raise a family and just tell you over and over again what an amazing job you are doing? Some of you will have that experience, but others have parents with their own strong views on how you should or should not be bringing up your children.

Oftentimes these opinions are well intentioned and come from a place of genuine love and support. Sometimes previous generations feel that different choices made by the next generation are somehow a judgement or negative comment on how they raised *you*. However, as a new parent there is really nothing harder than being told you are doing it "wrong," even if the critique is meant in the best way possible.

Discussing how you (and your partner) will handle this issue with your own families and each other's will prepare you for those tough conversations that may lie ahead.

Let me be the first to remind you: this is *your* baby. You get to raise them however you see best. And truly, dealing with tough family members is a great way to flex your advocacy skills, which is something all parents need to learn to use, as you are your child's only advocate for the first half of their life. This means you have to learn quickly how to stand up for them, even if doing so creates some discomfort for you.

NOTES ON QUESTION #6

CONCLUSION

I hope that the questions and exercises in this book have helped you feel more prepared for life beyond the birth of your little one. I also hope that you were able to plan and prepare in a way that felt easy and quick in the midst of the many preparations that you already have underway.

Before you close the book, I'd like to leave you with one final thought—a phrase really: Survival Mode. It's a phrase my therapist taught me when I was in the thick of postpartum depression and this phrase has carried my husband and I through job changes, house moves, the loss of my mother, my father moving in with us, a financial crisis, and more.

In our house, "survival mode" is a term we figuratively slap on life when things get rough and it helps us reset our expectations for a short time. "Survival mode" in our house means take out, more screen time for our kids, and a temporarily messy home. It's a way of acknowledging that we are in a rough patch and need to forgive ourselves a few things in order to just get through whatever is going on.

Think about what this term might mean for you so that when you bring your baby home you can allow yourselves the space you need to just survive for a while. Then, as life does that thing life does and throws tough stuff your way, you can gently place this phrase on any patch that requires you to just survive. The freedom that comes from forgiving yourself for more take out, more screen time, or whatever this phrase means to you can oftentimes give you the strength you need to power through.

Remember this: having a baby will be the best thing that ever happened to you, and it also may well be the hardest, scariest, most joyful, amazing, and horrible, wonderful experience of your life. It is filled with so many big feelings, some good and some hard.

Keeping your team strong is the key to navigating these new waters with confidence and joy.

Best wishes to you as you embark on the most wonderful, magical journey of your lives!

Kira

NOTES

NOTES

NOTES

NOTES

SUGGESTED READING

Cline, Foster and Jim Fay. *Love and Logic*, 2nd ed. Colorado Springs: NavPress, 2006.

Giordano, Suzy. *The Baby Sleep Solution*. New York: Penguin Group, 2006.

Gottman, John. *Raising an Emotionally Intelligent Child*. New York: Fireside, 1998.

Nelson, Ed.D., Jane. *Positive Discipline*. Ballantine Books: New York, 2006.

Sears, William and Martha Sears. *The Attachment Parenting Book: A Commonsense Guide to Understanding and Nurturing Your Baby*. Boston: Little, Brown and Company, 2001.

Sears, William, Martha Sears, Robert Sears, and James Sears. *The Baby Book*, 3rd ed. Boston: Little, Brown and Company, 2013.

Sears, William, Martha Sears, Robert Sears, and James Sears. *The Baby Sleep Book*. Boston: Little, Brown and Company, 2005.

West, Kim and Joanne Kenen. *The Sleep Lady's Good Night, Sleep Tight: Gentle Proven Solutions to Help Your Child Sleep Well and Wake Up Happy*, rev. ed. Cambridge, MA: Da Capo Press, 2009.

Weissbluth, M.D., Marc. *Healthy Sleep Habits, Happy Child*, 4th ed. New York: Ballantine Books, 2015.

ABOUT THE AUTHOR

Kira Dorrian has been working with expectant and new parents for the past decade as a childbirth educator, hypnotherapist, and parent coach. She is the co-creator of Future Focused Parenting, a parenting philosophy designed to take families from surviving to thriving. She is also the co-host of the podcast *Raising Adults: Future Focused Parenting*. Kira lives in Seattle with her husband and boy/girl twins. For more information on Kira and for additional, private coaching visit www.futurefocusedparenting.com.